THE AUTOIMMUNE PROTOCOL LIFESTYLE DIET

FLAVORFUL AND SAFE TO EAT RECIPES TO NOURISH YOUR BODY AND BOOST IMMUNE SYSTEM

322662362

Introduction To Autoimmune Protocol Diet

The immune system, also known as the autoimmune system, keeps you free of pathogens, fungi, and parasites that are designed to cause illness. It also keeps our body healthy when we are sick. The autoimmune system is designed to target foreign substances in your body and fight them off, keeping your body safe and healthy at all times. Because an autoimmune illness weakens or destroys the immune system, the body's primary defense mechanism is rendered ineffective. In an autoimmune illness, the immune system malfunctions and begins to assault healthy cells instead of foreign invaders. Among the many symptoms that this might bring on are inflammation and discomfort. What symptoms you experience ultimately contribute to your diagnosis. There are as many as eighty different types of autoimmune diseases. The symptoms of many of these diseases are similar, making diagnosis extremely challenging. In addition, multiple autoimmune diseases can coexist. Autoimmune diseases typically alternate between periods of remission (few or no symptoms) and flare-ups (worsening symptoms).

Every autoimmune disease has a set of specific criteria, or "markers," that must be met in order for a diagnosis to be made; some require blood work, while others are symptoms. If you don't meet the minimum number of markers required for a particular disease, you'll be told that your symptoms are non-specific and will have to wait to find out more about the condition. When you have an autoimmune disease, you can be extremely sick and unable to function, and you have all these symptoms that add up to... no one knows what it means. There are so many possible symptoms, and no two people have the same batch. It can take years, sometimes decades, to get a diagnosis. This can be extremely frustrating. Even though autoimmune diseases are very common, little is known about them and there are few effective treatments. They can impact practically every organ in the body and strike at any stage of life.

Role of Gut Health in Autoimmunity

The digestive tract is not just a system that breaks down food; it is also an important conduit between the outside world and the body's internal environment. Inside the gut is a diverse community of microorganisms called the gut microbiota, which is essential for immune system regulation, gut barrier integrity, and systemic inflammation control. A common observation in autoimmune diseases is dysbiosis, or an imbalance in the gut microbiota. This dysbiosis can result in increased intestinal permeability, also known as "leaky gut," where a compromised gut barrier allows harmful substances to enter the bloodstream, such as bacterial toxins and undigested food particles, which in turn triggers an immune response and promotes systemic inflammation. Dysbiosis can also upset the delicate balance of immune cells in the gut, which can cause abnormal immune activation and the start or worsening of autoimmune diseases.

Now let's take a look at a step by step breakdown of how gut health is important in guiding against unnecessary onset of immune disease or inflammatory symptoms in our body.

1. The trillions of bacteria, fungi, and other microorganisms that live in your gut are referred to as the gut microbiota
2. Balance is important, just as it is in a healthy community. When the balance of good and bad bacteria in your gut is disrupted, it can lead to problems. This disruption is called dysbiosis.
3. Your gut has a lining that acts as a barrier between the inside of your intestines and the rest of your body. It's like a protective wall that only allows certain things to pass through.
4. When there's dysbiosis, the gut barrier can become compromised, allowing unwanted substances like toxins and undigested food particles to "leak" through into your bloodstream. This is often referred to as leaky gut.

5. When these unwanted substances leak into the bloodstream, your immune system sees them as invaders and launches an attack. This immune response leads to inflammation throughout your body.
6. In some cases, this constant state of inflammation can confuse your immune system. Instead of just attacking invaders, it can start attacking your own tissues and organs, leading to autoimmune diseases.
7. Interestingly, the inflammation caused by autoimmunity can further disrupt the balance of the gut microbiota, creating a vicious cycle.

Basics of Autoimmune Protocol (AIP) Diet

People who suffer from autoimmune illnesses may find relief via the Autoimmune Protocol (AIP) diet, which aims to repair the gut, modify the immune system, and lower inflammation. It prioritizes nutrient-dense meals that promote healing and general health while avoiding those that may cause inflammation.

Important tenets of the AIP eating plan comprise:

Refined sugars, legumes, dairy, grains, processed oils, and nightshade vegetables are some of the most prevalent foods that cause inflammation.

Nutritionally dense foods should be prioritized, including fresh produce, lean meats, healthy fats, and fermented meals.

Supplements and therapeutic foods including digestive enzymes, collagen, probiotics, and bone broth are proven to promote gut health.

Benefits and Potential Risks

Many people have reported improvements in symptoms like joint pain, fatigue, digestive problems, and skin issues after following the AIP diet. Research has shown that dietary interventions, including the AIP diet, can modulate gut microbiota, reduce intestinal permeability, and attenuate inflammatory markers in patients with autoimmune conditions. But it's important to recognize that not everyone can follow the AIP diet, and that following restricted eating habits may come with hazards. The elimination phase may be difficult for some people to follow, which may result in feelings of deprivation and social isolation. Furthermore, the diet's restriction may make it difficult to achieve some dietary needs, such those for calcium and fiber, which, if left unchecked, may result in nutrient deficiencies. The AIP diet can be beneficial for many people, but it is not a one-size-fits-all approach, and tailored adjustments may be required depending on personal needs, preferences, and underlying medical conditions. It is advisable to speak with a qualified nutritionist or healthcare provider before beginning the AIP diet to ensure appropriate monitoring, guidance, and support along the way.

Getting Started with AIP

The Autoimmune Protocol (AIP) diet is a transformative journey that involves mental and emotional preparation in addition to a change in eating habits. It's important to set a solid foundation by organizing your pantry and fridge to make room for AIP-friendly foods before getting into the specifics of meal planning and ingredient substitutions.

Clearing Out Your Pantry and Fridge

1. Start by making a list of everything that is currently in your pantry, refrigerator, and freezer. This should include packaged foods, condiments, and spices in addition to perishables.
2. Get acquainted with the AIP diet's list of forbidden foods. Pay close attention to ingredient labels because a lot of packaged foods have inflammatory and hidden ingredients.
3. After you've determined which foods are off-limits, make a decision about whether to give them away to friends, food banks, or just throw them away. Keeping tempting foods that don't fit your dietary goals can lead to needless temptation and undermine your efforts.
4. Make a list of AIP-friendly foods to replenish your pantry and fridge.
5. To make your AIP journey go more smoothly, think about meal planning and batch cooking. Prepare meals and snacks ahead of time so you always have healthy options on hand for when hunger strikes
6. Accept the chance to experiment and discover new ingredients and recipes. In the kitchen, get inventive by adding AIP-compliant versions of your favorite recipes.

Adapting Family Favorites to AIP

Changing to an Autoimmune Protocol (AIP) diet doesn't have to mean saying goodbye to family favorites. With some creativity and resourcefulness, you can modify well-loved recipes to fit the AIP guidelines and keep meals wholesome and fulfilling for the entire family

- Learn about the main tenets of the AIP diet, such as which foods to include and which to avoid. By comprehending the reasoning behind these recommendations, you will be more prepared to make wise substitutions in family recipes

- Accept the bounty of naturally AIP-friendly, nutrient-dense whole foods: fruits, vegetables, high-quality proteins, healthy fats, herbs, and spices will serve as the building blocks of your modified recipes
- Try experimenting with AIP-friendly substitutes for common components. For example:

{Replace grains with cauliflower rice, sweet potato mash, or zucchini noodles.

Use homemade nut milks, coconut cream, or milk instead of dairy products.

For savory recipes, use coconut aminos for soy sauce.

Discover how versatile herbs and spices may be to enhance the taste and complexity of your food without having to use nightshades}

- Cooking methods should be modified to align with AIP guidelines. Roasting, steaming, sautéing, and slow cooking are examples of techniques that improve flavor and texture without using inflammatory ingredients.
- Invite your family members to participate in the process of adaptation by asking about their thoughts and preferences. Promote innovation and trial in the kitchen so that everyone enjoys helping to prepare meals together.
- When introducing adapted recipes to the family, open communication is essential. Be truthful about the modifications you've made, highlight the health advantages of AIP-friendly ingredients, and promote a willingness to try new flavors and textures.

A Comprehensive List of AIP-Friendly Foods

The Autoimmune Protocol (AIP) diet can be difficult to follow at first, but if you have access to a thorough list of foods that are allowed to be eaten, you'll be well-equipped to prepare wholesome, filling meals that promote your overall health and wellbeing.

1. Vegetables

Leafy greens (kale, spinach, Swiss chard)

Cruciferous vegetables (broccoli, cauliflower, Brussels sprouts)

Root vegetables (sweet potatoes, carrots, beets)

Squash (butternut squash, acorn squash, spaghetti squash)

Alliums (onions, garlic, leeks)

2. Fruits

Berries (strawberries, blueberries, raspberries)

Apples

Pears

Citrus fruits (lemons, limes, oranges)

Tropical fruits (mango, papaya, pineapple)

3. Quality Proteins

Grass-fed and pasture-raised meats (beef, lamb, pork)

Wild-caught fish (salmon, mackerel, sardines)

Free-range poultry (chicken, turkey, duck)

Organ meats (liver, heart, kidney)

Eggs (if tolerated)

4. Healthy Fats

Avocado

Coconut products (coconut oil, coconut milk, coconut cream)

Olives and extra virgin olive oil

Fatty fish (salmon, mackerel, herring)

Avocado oil

5. Herbs and Spices

Garlic

Ginger

Turmeric

Rosemary

Thyme

Cinnamon

6. Pantry Staples

Coconut aminos

Apple cider vinegar

Coconut flour

Arrowroot starch

Gelatin or collagen powder

Canned coconut milk

7. Gut-Healing Foods

Bone broth (homemade or store-bought)

Fermented vegetables (sauerkraut, kimchi)

Probiotic-rich foods (coconut yogurt, fermented pickles)

Digestive enzymes (supplement form)

Chapter 1: Breakfast and Brunch AIP Recipes

Sweet Potato Hash

Prep Time: 10 minutes
Cooking Time: 20 minutes
Serving Size: 4

Ingredients

2 medium sweet potatoes, peeled and diced

1/2 lb ground turkey or chicken

1 small onion, diced

2 cups fresh spinach

2 tablespoons coconut oil

1 teaspoon garlic powder

1 teaspoon dried thyme

1 teaspoon dried parsley

Salt to taste

Cooking Instructions

Heat the coconut oil in a large skillet over medium heat. Add the diced sweet potatoes and cook for 5 to 7 minutes, or until they begin to soften. Next, add the ground turkey or chicken to the skillet, breaking it up with a spatula, and cook until browned. Cook for another 3 to 4 minutes, or until the onion is translucent. Finally, add the fresh spinach and cook until it wilts.

Finally, sprinkle the mixture with the salt, garlic powder, thyme, and parsley. Stir to mix. Cook for a further two to three minutes, or until everything is thoroughly heated and incorporated.

Nutritional Values (per serving):
Calories: 240 kcal, Protein: 15g, Carbs: 20g, Fat: 11g, Fiber: 4g, Sugar: 5g

Coconut Flour Pancakes

Prep Time: 10 minutes
Cooking Time: 15 minutes
Serving Size: 4

Ingredients

1/2 cup coconut flour

2 ripe bananas, mashed

1/2 cup coconut milk

2 eggs (optional, omit if not tolerated)

Coconut oil for cooking

Fresh berries for serving

Honey or maple syrup (in moderation, optional)

Cooking Instructions

Put the coconut flour, mashed bananas, coconut milk, and eggs (if using) in a mixing bowl and mix until smooth and well combined. You can add a little more coconut milk if the batter is too thick. Heat a non-stick skillet or griddle over medium heat and brush it lightly with coconut oil. For each pancake, pour about 1/4 cup of batter onto the skillet. Continue cooking the remaining batter, adding extra coconut oil to the skillet as needed, and cook the pancakes for another one to two minutes on each side, until bubbles form on the surface and the pan is golden brown.

Serve the pancakes hot, garnished with fresh berries and, if desired, a drizzle of honey or maple syrup (in moderation).

Nutritional Values (per serving, without toppings):
Calories: 180 kcal, Protein: 5g, Carbs: 20g, Fat: 9g, Fiber: 6g, Sugar: 7g

Zucchini Noodles with Pesto

Prep Time: 15 minutes
Cooking Time: 5 minutes
Serving Size: 4

For the zucchini noodles:

4 medium zucchinis

1 cup cherry tomatoes, sliced

1/2 cup black olives, sliced

For the AIP-friendly pesto:

2 cups fresh basil leaves

2 cloves garlic, minced

1/4 cup extra virgin olive oil

1/4 cup pumpkin seeds (or pine nuts)

Salt to taste

Cooking Instructions

Using a spiralizer or julienne peeler, thinly slice the zucchini into noodles and set aside. In a food processor or blender, add the minced garlic, olive oil, pumpkin seeds (or pine nuts), and a pinch of salt. Blend until smooth, stopping occasionally to scrape down the sides. Heat a small amount of olive oil in a large skillet over medium heat. Add the zucchini noodles and cook for two to three minutes, or until just tender.

After taking the skillet off of the burner, toss the zucchini noodles in the homemade pesto until well coated. Transfer the noodles to serving dishes and garnish with the black olives and cherry tomatoes slices.

Nutritional Values (per serving):
Calories: 180 kcal, Protein: 5g, Carbs: 10g, Fat: 15g, Fiber: 4g, Sugar: 4g

Chicken and Vegetable Stir-Fry

Prep Time: 10 minutes
Cooking Time: 15 minutes
Serving Size: 4

Ingredients

2 boneless, skinless chicken breasts, shredded

2 cups mixed vegetables (broccoli florets, sliced carrots, diced bell peppers)

3 tablespoons coconut aminos

2 cloves garlic, minced

2 tablespoons coconut oil

Salt to taste

Cauliflower rice for serving

Cooking Instructions

Heat the coconut oil in a large skillet or wok over medium-high heat. Add the minced garlic and sauté for 1 minute, or until fragrant. Add the shredded chicken breast and cook, stirring, for 5 to 6 minutes, or until lightly browned. Add the mixed vegetables and stir-fry for 4 to 5 minutes, or until they begin to soften but remain crisp. Cook for a further two to three minutes, or until everything is heated through and well combined. Season with salt to taste. Serve the chicken and vegetable stir-fry over cauliflower rice and drizzle with coconut aminos; stir to coat the chicken and vegetables evenly.

Nutritional Values (per serving, without cauliflower rice):

Calories: 180 kcal, Protein: 20g, Carbs: 10g, Fat: 7g, Fiber: 3g, Sugar: 4g

Berry Smoothie Bowl

Prep Time: 5 minutes
Serving Size: 1

Ingredients

1 cup mixed berries (such as strawberries, blueberries, and raspberries), fresh or frozen

1/2 cup coconut milk

1 scoop collagen powder (optional)

1 ripe banana, sliced

2 tablespoons shredded coconut

AIP-friendly granola made from seeds and dried fruit (store-bought or homemade)

Cooking Instructions

Mix the berries, coconut milk, and collagen powder (if using) in a blender and process until smooth. Transfer the smoothie into a bowl and garnish with banana slices, shredded coconut, and AIP-compliant granola.

Nutritional Values (per serving, without granola):
Calories: 250 kcal, Protein: 5g, Carbs: 30g, Fat: 14g, Fiber: 8g, Sugar: 15g

Turmeric Scrambled Eggs

Prep Time: 10 minutes
Cooking Time: 10 minutes
Serving Size: 2

Ingredients

4 eggs (optional, omit if not tolerated)

1/2 teaspoon ground turmeric

1 cup chopped spinach

1/2 cup diced cooked sweet potatoes

2 tablespoons coconut oil

Salt to taste

Sliced avocado for serving

Fresh cilantro for garnish

Cooking Instructions

Whisk the eggs and ground turmeric together thoroughly in a mixing bowl. Heat the coconut oil in a skillet over medium heat. Add the diced sweet potatoes and chopped spinach to the skillet. Cook for two to three minutes, or until the sweet potatoes are heated through. Pour the whisked eggs into the skillet with the sweet potatoes and spinach. Cook, stirring occasionally, until the eggs are scrambled and cooked to your desired consistency. Season with salt to taste.

Serve the scrambled eggs hot with sliced avocado and a sprinkle of fresh cilantro.

Nutritional Values (per serving, without avocado):
Calories: 250 kcal, Protein: 11g, Carbs: 10g, Fat: 19g, Fiber: 3g, Sugar: 2g

AIP Breakfast Skillet

Prep Time: 10 minutes
Cooking Time: 20 minutes
Serving Size: 4

Ingredients

1 lb ground turkey or pork sausage

2 medium sweet potatoes, peeled and diced

1 small onion, diced

2 cups kale, chopped

2 tablespoons extra virgin olive oil

1 avocado, sliced

Salt to taste

Cooking Instructions

In a cast-iron skillet set over medium heat, add 1 tablespoon of olive oil. Add the ground turkey or pork sausage and cook, breaking it up with a spatula, until it is browned. Remove the cooked meat from the skillet and set it aside. Repeat with the remaining tablespoon of olive oil in the same skillet. Add the diced sweet potatoes and cook for 5 to 7 minutes, or until they begin to soften. Add the diced onion and cook for an additional 3 to 4 minutes, or until the onion is translucent. Stir in the chopped kale and cook until it wilts. Return the cooked meat to the skillet and mix everything together.

Season with salt to taste. Top the skillet with avocado slices and drizzle with a little extra virgin olive oil before serving.

Nutritional Values (per serving):
Calories: 380 kcal, Protein: 25g, Carbs: 20g, Fat: 24g, Fiber: 6g, Sugar: 4g

Smoked Salmon and Avocado Wrap

Prep Time: 10 minutes
Serving Size: 4

Ingredients

4 large collard green leaves

4 oz smoked salmon

1 ripe avocado, thinly sliced

1 cup shredded lettuce

Toothpicks for securing

For the dipping sauce:

2 tablespoons coconut aminos

1 teaspoon grated ginger

Cooking Instructions

Rinse the collard greens, pat dry with paper towels, trim off the tough stems, and lay flat on a cutting board. Evenly distribute the avocado slices, shredded lettuce, and smoked salmon among the leaves, centering them in each one. Each collard green leaf should be folded over the filling and tightly rolled up like a burrito, securing with toothpicks if necessary. Meanwhile, make the dipping sauce by whisking together the grated ginger and coconut aminos in a small bowl. Serve the wraps with the dipping sauce on the side.

Nutritional Values (per serving):
Calories: 150 kcal, Protein: 10g, Carbs: 6g, Fat: 10gz, Fiber: 4g, Sugar: 1g

Plantain Waffles

Prep Time: 10 minutes
Cooking Time: 15 minutes
Serving Size: 4

Ingredients

2 ripe plantains, mashed

1/2 cup coconut flour

1/4 cup coconut oil, melted

1/2 cup coconut milk

Coconut oil or cooking spray for greasing the waffle iron

Coconut yogurt and fresh fruit for topping

Cooking Instructions

Preheat your waffle iron as directed by the manufacturer. In a mixing bowl, combine mashed plantains, coconut flour, melted coconut oil, and coconut milk. Mix until smooth and well combined. Once the waffle iron is heated, lightly grease it with coconut oil or cooking spray. Pour enough batter onto the waffle iron to cover the surface. Close the lid and cook the waffles according to the manufacturer's instructions. When the waffles are golden brown and crispy, carefully remove them from the waffle iron and transfer them to a plate. Before serving, top the waffles with coconut yogurt and fresh fruit.

Nutritional Values (per serving, without toppings):
Calories: 250 kcal, Protein: 3g, Carbs: 30g, Fat: 14g, Fiber: 5g, Sugar: 12g

Cauliflower Breakfast Bowl

Prep Time: 10 minutes
Cooking Time: 20-25 minutes
Serving Size: 2

Ingredients

1 small head cauliflower, cut into florets

4 slices bacon, chopped

1 cup sliced mushrooms

2 cups arugula

Balsamic glaze (without added sugar)

Cooking Instructions

Adjust the oven temperature to 400°F (200°C). Transfer the chopped bacon, sliced mushrooms, and cauliflower florets to a parchment paper-lined baking sheet. Roast for 20 to 25 minutes, or until the bacon is crispy and the cauliflower is golden brown. Meanwhile, divide the arugula among serving bowls. After the arugula is roasted, spoon the bacon, mushroom, and cauliflower mixture over it. Drizzle with sugar-free balsamic glaze, to taste.

Nutritional Values (per serving):
Calories: 250 kcal, Protein: 12g, Carbs: 12g, Fat: 18g, Fiber: 5g, Sugar: 5g

AIP Breakfast Casserole

Prep Time: 20 minutes
Cooking Time: 25-30 minutes
Serving Size: 6

Ingredients

1 lb ground beef or turkey, cooked and drained

2 medium sweet potatoes, peeled and thinly sliced

2 cups mixed vegetables (such as bell peppers, onions, and spinach), sautéed

8 eggs (optional, omit if not tolerated)

1 teaspoon dried herbs (such as parsley, thyme, or basil)

Salt and pepper to taste

Cooking Instructions

Set your oven to 375°F (190°C). Grease a baking dish with coconut oil or olive oil. Transfer the cooked ground beef or turkey to the bottom of the dish in an even layer. Top the meat with a layer of thinly sliced sweet potatoes. Finally, cover the sweet potatoes with the sautéed mixed vegetables. Whisk the eggs (if using) with the salt, pepper, and dried herbs in a mixing bowl. Pour the egg mixture evenly over the casserole, covering all the ingredients. Bake in the preheated oven for 25 to 30 minutes, or until the edges are golden brown and the eggs are set. Take the casserole out of the oven and allow it to cool slightly before slicing and serving.

Nutritional Values (per serving):
Calories: 280 kcal, Protein: 20g, Carbs: 15g, Fat: 15g, Fiber: 3, Sugar: 4g

Turmeric Coconut Porridge

Prep Time: 5 minutes
Cooking Time: 15 minutes
Serving Size: 2

Ingredients

2 cups coconut milk

1/2 cup shredded coconut

2 ripe bananas, mashed

1 teaspoon ground turmeric

Sliced bananas and cinnamon for serving

Cooking Instructions

Coconut milk, shredded coconut, mashed bananas, and ground turmeric should all be combined in a saucepan and brought to a gentle simmer over medium-low heat. After that, reduce the heat to low and simmer the porridge, stirring occasionally, until it thickens to the desired consistency, about 10 to 15 minutes. After that, remove the pot from the heat and allow it to cool slightly before serving it warm, garnished with sliced bananas and cinnamon.

Nutritional Values (per serving, without toppings):
Calories: 320 kcal, Protein: 3g, Carbs: 20g, Fat: 27g, Fiber: 5g, Sugar: 12g

Chicken and Vegetable Frittata

Prep Time: 10 minutes
Cooking Time: 20-25 minutes
Serving Size: 4

Ingredients

6 eggs (optional, omit if not tolerated)

1 cup diced cooked chicken

1 cup chopped spinach

1 cup sliced mushrooms

Coconut oil for greasing

Salt and pepper to taste (optional, omit for strict AIP)

Cooking Instructions

Heat a greased skillet over medium heat on the stovetop. Pour the egg mixture into the skillet and spread it evenly. Preheat your oven to 350°F (175°C). In a mixing bowl, beat together the eggs (if using) until well beaten. Stir in diced cooked chicken, chopped spinach, and sliced mushrooms. Season with salt and pepper. (omit for strict AIP). Cook for 3–4 minutes, or until the edges begin to set. Transfer the skillet to the preheated oven and bake for 15-20 minutes, or until the frittata is fully set and slightly golden on top. Remove from the skillet and let cool for a few minutes before slicing; serve with a side of mixed greens.

Nutritional Values (per serving, without optional ingredients):
Calories: 180 kcal, Protein: 20g, Carbs: 3g, Fat: 10g, Fiber: 1g, Sugar: 1g

AIP Breakfast Burrito Bowl

Prep Time: 10 minutes
Cooking Time: 10 minutes
Serving Size: 2

Ingredients

2 cups cauliflower rice

1 cup shredded chicken (cooked without any non-AIP ingredients)

1 ripe avocado, diced

1 cucumber, sliced

Lime juice for drizzling

Chopped fresh herbs like cilantro and mint for garnish

Salt to taste

Cooking Instructions

If not already done, prepare the cauliflower rice by either purchasing it already riced or pulsing the cauliflower florets in a food processor until they resemble rice. Heat a skillet over medium heat, add the cauliflower rice, and cook, stirring occasionally, until the cauliflower is tender, 5 to 7 minutes. Meanwhile, arrange the shredded chicken, diced avocado, and sliced cucumber in serving bowls. After the cauliflower rice is cooked, divide it among the serving bowls, top with chopped fresh herbs, squeeze some lime juice over each, and season with salt to taste.

Nutritional Values (per serving):
Calories: 300 kcal, Protein: 20g, Carbs: 15g, Fat: 18g, Fiber: 10g, Sugar: 3g

Baked Apples with Cinnamon

Prep Time: 10 minutes
Cooking Time: 25-30 minutes
Serving Size: 4

Ingredients

4 medium apples

1/4 cup chopped nuts (such as walnuts or pecans)

1/4 cup shredded coconut

1 teaspoon cinnamon

Coconut yogurt for serving

Cooking Instructions

Preheat your oven to 350°F (175°C). Set aside the apples to cool in a baking dish after coring them. In a small bowl, combine the chopped nuts, shredded coconut, and cinnamon. Gently stuff each cored apple with the nut and coconut mixture. Cover the baking dish with aluminum foil and bake in the preheated oven for 25 to 30 minutes, or until the apples are tender. Remove from the oven and let cool slightly before serving. Serve the baked apples warm with a dollop of coconut yogurt on top.

Chapter 2: Snacks and Sweets AIP Recipes

Baked Sweet Potato Chips

Prep Time: 10 minutes
Cooking Time: 20-25 minutes
Serving Size: 4

Ingredients

2 medium sweet potatoes, thinly sliced

2 tablespoons coconut oil, melted

Sea salt to taste

Cooking Instructions

Set aside a baking sheet lined with parchment paper, preheat your oven to 375°F (190°C), wash and peel your sweet potatoes, and then use a mandoline slicer or a sharp knife to thinly slice them into rounds. Transfer the sliced sweet potatoes to a large bowl and toss them with melted coconut oil until well coated. Arrange your sweet potato slices in a single layer, being careful not to overlap, on the prepared baking sheet. Dredge the sweet potato slices in sea salt; bake in the preheated oven for 20 to 25 minutes, rotating the chips halfway through, until they become crispy and golden brown. Take the chips out of the oven and allow them to cool for a short while before serving.

Nutritional Values (per serving):
Calories: 120 kcal, Protein: 1g, Carbs: 15g, Fat: 7, Fiber: 2g, Sugar: 3g

Coconut Berry Bliss Balls

Prep Time: 10 minutes
Serving Size: 12 bliss balls

Ingredients

1 cup unsweetened shredded coconut

1/2 cup mixed berries (such as strawberries, blueberries, or raspberries), fresh or thawed if frozen

1/4 cup coconut butter

1 tablespoon honey (optional, omit if not tolerated)

1/2 teaspoon vanilla extract (optional, omit if not tolerated)

Pinch of sea salt

Cooking Instructions

Shredded coconut, mixed berries, coconut butter, honey, vanilla extract, and a small pinch of sea salt should all be combined in a food processor and pulsed until a thick dough forms. Using your hands, roll the dough into small balls that are about 1 inch in diameter. To firm up, place the bliss balls on a baking sheet lined with parchment paper and refrigerate for at least half an hour. Once firm, store the bliss balls in the refrigerator in an airtight container until you're ready to serve.

Nutritional Values (per serving, based on 1 bliss ball):
Calories: 70 kcal, Protein: 1g, Carbs: 5g, Fat: 6g, Fiber: 2g, Sugar: 3g

Cucumber Avocado Boats

Prep Time: 10 minutes
Serving Size: 4

Ingredients

2 large cucumbers

1 ripe avocado

1/2 lemon, juiced

1/4 cup diced red bell pepper

1/4 cup diced cucumber (from the scooped out center)

1 tablespoon chopped fresh cilantro

Salt to taste

Cooking Instructions

Slice the cucumbers lengthwise in half, then remove the seeds to form "boats". In a bowl, mash the avocado with the lemon juice until it becomes smooth. Add the diced red bell pepper, diced cucumber, chopped cilantro, and salt to taste. Evenly fill each cucumber boat with the avocado mixture.

Nutritional Values (per serving):
Calories: 90 kcal, Protein: 2g, Carbs: 7g, Fat: 7g, Fiber: 4g, Sugar: 2g

AIP Trail Mix

Prep Time: 5 minutes
Serving Size: 8

Ingredients

1 cup unsweetened coconut flakes

1/2 cup sliced or chopped dried fruit (such as unsweetened dried mango, apple, or banana)

1/2 cup raw pumpkin seeds (pepitas)

1/2 cup raw sunflower seeds

1/4 cup dried cranberries (look for ones sweetened with apple juice or omit if preferred)

1/4 cup raw or lightly toasted coconut chips

1/4 teaspoon sea salt

Cooking Instructions

To ensure even distribution of ingredients, combine all the ingredients in a large mixing bowl and toss well. Store the trail mix in an airtight container until you're ready to serve it or pack it for snacks.

Nutritional Values (per serving, approximately 1/4 cup):
Calories: 180 kcal, Protein: 4g, Carbs: 15g, Fat: 12g, Fiber: 4g, Sugar: 8g

Baked Cinnamon Apples

Prep Time: 10 minutes
Cooking Time: 35-40 minutes
Serving Size: 4

Ingredients

4 medium-sized apples, cored and sliced

1 teaspoon ground cinnamon

1 tablespoon coconut oil, melted

1 tablespoon honey or maple syrup (optional, omit for strict AIP)

1/4 cup water

Cooking Instructions

Set the oven to 350°F (175°C). In a bowl, combine the sliced apples, melted coconut oil, ground cinnamon, and honey or maple syrup (if desired). Make sure the apples are well coated. Transfer the apple slices to a baking dish and cover the apples with water. Place aluminum foil over the baking dish and bake in the preheated oven for 25 to 30 minutes, stirring the apples halfway through. After that, take off the foil and bake for a further 5 to 10 minutes to allow the liquid to slightly reduce.

Nutritional Values (per serving):
Calories: 100 kcal, Protein: 0g, Carbs: 25g, Fat: 3g, Fiber: 4g, Sugar: 19g

Chapter 3: Vegetarian and Vegan AIP Recipes

Roasted Sweet Potato and Kale Salad

Prep Time: 10 minutes
Cooking Time: 25 minutes
Serving Size: 4

Ingredients

2 medium sweet potatoes, peeled and cubed

4 cups kale, stems removed and torn into bite-sized pieces

2 tablespoons olive oil

Salt to taste

For the Lemon-Tahini Dressing:

1/4 cup tahini

2 tablespoons lemon juice

1 tablespoon apple cider vinegar

1 clove garlic, minced

2-3 tablespoons water (adjust for desired consistency)

Salt to taste

Cooking Instructions

Set the oven to 400°F (200°C). Take a baking sheet, add some olive oil, sprinkle some salt on it, and toss to coat it evenly. Roast the sweet potatoes for 20 to 25 minutes, or until they are soft and lightly browned, turning them over halfway through. In the meantime, prepare the kale by putting it in a big bowl, drizzling it with some olive oil and salt, and massaging it with your hands for a few minutes until it softens. Whisk together the tahini, lemon juice, apple cider vinegar, minced garlic, and water in a small bowl until smooth. Season with salt to taste. When the sweet potatoes are done roasting, let them cool slightly. To assemble the salad, place the massaged kale in a serving bowl or platter, top with the roasted sweet potatoes, and drizzle with the lemon-tahini dressing.

Nutritional Values (per serving):
Calories: 250 kcal, Protein: 5g, Carbs: 25g, Fat: 15g, Fiber: 5g, Sugar: 4g

Cauliflower Rice Stir-Fry

Prep Time: 10 minutes
Cooking Time: 15 minutes
Serving Size: 4

Ingredients

1 head cauliflower, riced (or 4 cups pre-riced cauliflower)

1 bell pepper, thinly sliced

1 carrot, thinly sliced

1 cup broccoli florets

2 tablespoons coconut aminos

2 cloves garlic, minced

2 tablespoons coconut oil

Salt to taste

Optional: chopped green onions for garnish

Cooking Instructions

In a big skillet or wok over medium heat, heat the coconut oil. Add the minced garlic and sauté for about 1 minute until fragrant. Add the bell pepper, carrot, and broccoli florets, and stir-fry for about 5-7 minutes, or until the vegetables are soft and crisp.

Add the riced cauliflower and cook, stirring frequently, for an additional 3–4 minutes, or until the cauliflower is cooked through but still slightly firm. Add coconut aminos to the cauliflower rice and vegetable mixture, stir to mix, and cook for an additional two to three minutes to let the flavors meld. Taste and adjust the seasoning. Take off the heat and serve hot, topped with finely chopped green onions.

Nutritional Values (per serving):
Calories: 100 kcal, Protein: 3g, Carbs: 12g, Fat: 6g, Fiber: 4g, Sugar: 5g

Noodles with Pesto

Prep Time: 15 minutes
Cooking Time: 5 minutes
Serving Size: 4

Ingredients

4 medium zucchinis, spiralized into noodles

1 ripe avocado

1 cup fresh basil leaves

2 cloves garlic, minced

2 tablespoons olive oil

Salt to taste

Optional toppings: chopped fresh tomatoes, sliced black olives, pine nuts (if tolerated)

Cooking Instructions

To make the avocado pesto, place the avocado, minced garlic, basil leaves, olive oil, and a small pinch of salt in a blender or food processor and process until smooth and creamy. In a large skillet, heat a small amount of olive oil over medium heat. Add the zucchini noodles and cook, tossing occasionally, for two to three minutes, or until they are soft but still have a slight crunch. After the zucchini noodles are cooked, take them off the heat and place them in a serving bowl.

Drizzle the avocado pesto over the noodles and toss to coat them thoroughly. If preferred, garnish the dish with additional toppings.

Nutritional Values (per serving, without optional toppings):
Calories: 150 kcal, Protein: 3g, Carbs: 10g, Fat: 12g, Fiber: 5g, Sugar: 4g

Portobello Mushroom Burgers

Prep Time: 10 minutes
Cooking Time: 10-14 minutes
Serving Size: 4

Ingredients

4 large portobello mushrooms, stems removed

1 avocado, sliced

1 roasted red pepper, sliced

4 large lettuce leaves

Salt to taste

Optional: AIP-friendly sauce (e.g., homemade olive oil and lemon dressing)

Cooking Instructions

Turn the heat up to medium-high. Wipe off any dirt from the portobello mushrooms with a damp cloth. Drizzle both sides with a little olive oil and season with salt. Put the mushrooms, gill-side down, on the grill and cook for 5 to 7 minutes on each side, or until they are soft and have grill marks. Prepare the lettuce leaves on serving plates while the mushrooms are grilling. When the mushrooms are done, place them on top of the lettuce leaves. Garnish each mushroom with sliced avocado and roasted red peppers. Serve, with the option to drizzle with sauce that is suitable for the AIP.

Nutritional Values (per serving):
Calories: 100 kcal, Protein: 3g, Carbs: 8g, Fat: 7g, Fiber: 4g, Sugar: 2g

Stuffed Bell Peppers

Prep Time: 15 minutes
Cooking Time: 40-45 minutes
Serving Size: 4 servings

Ingredients

4 large bell peppers (any color), halved and seeds removed

2 cups cauliflower rice

1 cup cooked lentils or chickpeas (if tolerated)

1 small onion, diced

2 cloves garlic, minced

1 tablespoon coconut oil

1 teaspoon dried oregano

1 teaspoon dried basil

Salt to taste

Fresh parsley, chopped (for garnish)

Cooking Instructions

A large skillet should be heated to 375°F (190°C). In the skillet, add the minced garlic and diced onion and sauté for 3–4 minutes, or until the onion is softened. Next, add the cauliflower rice and cook for another 5–7 minutes, or until it is tender. Finally, add the cooked lentils or chickpeas, dried oregano, dried basil, and salt to taste.

Cook for a further 2–3 minutes, or until the flavors meld. Lay out the cut side up bell pepper halves in a baking dish. Spoon the cauliflower rice mixture into each half, gently pressing to pack it in. Cover the baking dish with foil and bake in the preheated oven for 25 to 30 minutes, or until the bell peppers are soft. Then, take off the foil and bake for a further 5 to 10 minutes to lightly brown the tops. Before serving, garnish with fresh parsley that has been chopped.

Nutritional Values (per serving):
Calories: 220 kcal, Protein: 10g, Carbs: 30g, Fat: 6g, Fiber: 10g, Sugar: 10g

Butternut Squash Soup

Prep Time: 15 minutes
Cooking Time: 25 minutes
Serving Size: 4

Ingredients

1 medium butternut squash, peeled, seeded, and diced

1 can (13.5 oz) coconut milk

1 tablespoon fresh ginger, grated

1 teaspoon ground turmeric

4 cups bone broth or vegetable broth

Salt to taste

Fresh herbs (such as parsley or cilantro) for garnish

Cooking Instructions

Diced butternut squash, coconut milk, grated ginger, ground turmeric, and broth should all be combined in a large pot. Heat the mixture to a boil over medium-high heat, then lower the heat and simmer until the butternut squash is tender, about 20 to 25 minutes. Puree the soup with an immersion blender or regular blender until it's smooth and creamy, and then serve hot, garnished with fresh herbs.

Nutritional Values (per serving):

Calories: 220 kcal, Protein: 4g, Carbs: 25g, Fat: 14, Fiber: 5g, Sugar: 6g

Crispy Baked Plantain Chips

Prep Time: 10 minutes
Cooking Time: 15-20 minutes
Serving Size: 4

Ingredients

2 green plantains

2 tablespoons coconut oil, melted

Sea salt to taste

Guacamole or salsa for serving (optional)

Cooking Instructions

Set aside a large bowl, toss the plantain slices with melted coconut oil until evenly coated, then arrange the slices in a single layer, making sure they are not overlapping, on the prepared baking sheet. Preheat your oven to 375°F (190°C). Peel and thinly slice the plantains using a sharp knife or mandoline slicer. Sprinkle the plantain slices with sea salt to taste. Bake in the preheated oven for 15-20 minutes, flipping halfway through. When the plantain chips are crispy and golden brown, remove from the oven and allow to cool for a few minutes before serving. You can serve the crispy baked plantain chips with salsa or guacamole, if you'd like.

Nutritional Values (per serving, without dip):
Calories: 120 kcal, Protein: 1g, Carbs: 20g, Fat: 5g, Fiber: 2g, Sugar: 8g

Cabbage Rolls with Cauliflower Rice

Prep Time: 30 minutes
Cooking Time: 50 minutes
Serving Size: 4

Ingredients

1 head of cabbage

1 small head of cauliflower

1 cup mushrooms, finely chopped

1 small onion, finely chopped

2 cloves garlic, minced

1 teaspoon dried thyme

1 teaspoon dried oregano

Salt to taste

1 can (14 oz) AIP-friendly tomato sauce

1 cup bone broth or water

Fresh parsley, chopped (for garnish)

Cooking Instructions

Cut the cauliflower into florets and pulse in a food processor until it resembles rice. Preheat the oven to 350°F (175°C). Bring a large pot of water to a boil. Carefully remove the outer leaves of the cabbage and blanch them in the boiling water for two to three minutes, until softened. Set aside to cool.

Add the chopped onions, garlic, and mushrooms to a skillet over medium heat. Cook until the ingredients soften, about 5 minutes. Add the cauliflower "rice" to the skillet and cook for an additional 5 minutes. Stir in the dried oregano and dried thyme, and adjust with salt to taste. Take the skillet off the heat. Spoon a spoonful of the cauliflower mixture onto each cabbage leaf. Roll the cabbage leaf up, tucking in the sides as you roll. Place seam side down in a baking dish. After combining the tomato sauce, bone broth, or water in a bowl, pour the mixture over the cabbage rolls in the baking dish, cover with aluminum foil, and bake in the preheated oven for 45 to 50 minutes, or until the rolls are tender. Before serving, sprinkle the rolls with chopped parsley.

Nutritional Values (per serving):
Calories: 180 kcal, Protein: 6g, Carbs: 25g, Fat: 6g, Fiber: 9g, Sugar: 12g

Coconut Curry Veggie Stir-Fry

Prep Time: 10 minutes
Cooking Time: 15 minutes
Serving Size: 4

Ingredients

2 tablespoons coconut oil

4 cups mixed vegetables (such as bell peppers, broccoli, carrots, snap peas)

2 cloves garlic, minced

1 teaspoon minced ginger

1 teaspoon curry powder (AIP-friendly blend)

1/2 teaspoon turmeric powder

1/2 cup coconut milk

Salt to taste

Fresh cilantro for garnish (optional)

Cooking Instructions

In a large skillet or wok over medium heat, heat the coconut oil. Add the minced garlic and ginger and sauté for 1 minute, or until fragrant. Add the mixed vegetables to the skillet and stir-fry for 5 to 7 minutes, or until they are crisp-tender.

Sprinkle the vegetables with curry powder and turmeric powder and stir to coat them evenly. After adding the coconut milk to the skillet and thoroughly mixing, cook the vegetables for two to three more minutes, or until they are heated through. Season with salt and, if preferred, garnish with fresh cilantro.

Nutritional Values (per serving):
Calories: 120 kcal, Protein: 2g, Carbs: 10g, Fat: 9g, Fiber: 3g, Sugar: 4g

Baked Acorn Squash with Cinnamon

Prep Time: 10 minutes
Cooking Time: 35-50 minutes
Serving Size: 4

Ingredients

2 acorn squash, halved and seeds removed

Cinnamon (AIP-friendly)

Cooking Instructions

After preheating the oven to 400°F (200°C), place the cut side down acorn squash halves on a baking sheet lined with parchment paper. Bake the squash for 30 to 40 minutes, or until it is tender and pierces easily with a fork. Once the squash is done, remove it from the oven and carefully turn it over so the cut side is now facing up. Scatter the exposed flesh of the squash with the cinnamon, then return it to the oven and bake for a further 5 to 10 minutes, letting the cinnamon seep into the squash. After that, take it out of the oven and allow it to cool slightly before serving.

Nutritional Values (per serving):
Calories: 80 kcal, Protein: 1g, Carbs: 20g, Fat: 0g, Fiber: 4g, Sugar: 0g

Mashed Turnips with Herbs

Prep Time: 10 minutes
Cooking Time: 20 minutes
Serving Size: 4

Ingredients

4 medium turnips, peeled and diced

2 cloves garlic, minced

1/4 cup coconut milk

2 tablespoons fresh parsley or chives, chopped

Salt to taste

Cooking Instructions

Turnips should be diced and placed in a pot with water to cover. Turnips should be brought to a boil over medium-high heat, then simmered for 15 to 20 minutes, or until fork-tender. Once the turnips are cooked, they should be drained and put back in the pot along with chopped fresh herbs, minced garlic, and coconut milk. Mash the turnips with a potato masher or fork until the desired consistency is reached. Add a little more coconut milk if the mixture is too thick. Season to taste and stir to combine. Serve hot, garnished with extra fresh herbs.

Nutritional Values (per serving):
Calories: 70 kcal, Protein: 2g, Carbs: 10g, Fat: 3g, Fiber: 3g, Sugar: 5g

Grilled Eggplant with Balsamic Glaze

Prep Time: 10 minutes
Cooking Time: 10-15 minutes
Serving Size: 4

Ingredients

1 large eggplant, sliced into rounds

2 tablespoons extra virgin olive oil

Salt to taste

1/2 cup balsamic vinegar

Fresh basil leaves for garnish

Cooking Instructions

Preheat the grill to medium-high heat. Brush the eggplant slices on both sides with olive oil and season with salt. Grill the eggplant slices for 3–4 minutes on each side, or until they are soft and caramelized; depending on the size of your grill, you may need to cook them in batches. While the eggplant is grilling, make the balsamic glaze. In a small saucepan, bring the vinegar to a simmer over medium heat. Cook for 5-7 minutes, stirring occasionally, until the vinegar has reduced by half and has a syrupy consistency. When the eggplant is perfectly grilled, remove it from the grill and place it on a serving platter. Drizzle the grilled eggplant slices with the balsamic glaze. Garnish with fresh basil leaves.

Nutritional Values (per serving):
Calories: 90 kcal, Protein: 1g, Carbs: 12g, Fat: 4g, Fiber: 4g, Sugar: 7g

Cauliflower Mashed Potatoes

Prep Time: 10 minutes
Cooking Time: 10 minutes
Serving Size: 4

Ingredients

1 medium head of cauliflower, chopped into florets

1/4 cup coconut milk

2 cloves garlic, minced

2 tablespoons nutritional yeast

Salt to taste

Cooking Instructions

Steam the cauliflower until the florets are tender, 8 to 10 minutes. Then, transfer the steamed cauliflower to a food processor or blender. Add the coconut milk, nutritional yeast, minced garlic, and a pinch of salt. Blend until smooth and creamy, adding more coconut milk to reach the desired consistency. Taste and adjust the seasoning. Serve hot as a tasty and healthy substitute for mashed potatoes.

Nutritional Values (per serving):
Calories: 70 kcal, Protein: 3g, Carbs: 9g, Fat: 3g, Fiber: 4g, Sugar: 3g

Spinach and Mushroom Avocado Dressing

Prep Time: 10 minutes
Serving Size: 4

Ingredients

6 cups fresh spinach leaves

1 cup sliced mushrooms

1 ripe avocado

2 tablespoons fresh lemon juice

2 tablespoons extra virgin olive oil

Salt to taste

Optional toppings: sliced radishes, shredded carrots, or diced cucumber

Cooking Instructions

Fresh spinach leaves and sliced mushrooms should be combined in a large mixing bowl. In a small bowl, mash the ripe avocado with a fork until smooth. Add fresh lemon juice, extra virgin olive oil, and a pinch of salt to the mashed avocado, and mix until well combined to make the dressing. Pour the avocado dressing over the spinach and mushroom mixture, tossing gently to coat the salad evenly.

Divide the salad onto serving plates, and garnish with desired toppings.

Nutritional Values (per serving):
Calories: 150 kcal, Protein: 3g, Carbs: 9g, Fat: 12g, Fiber: 5g, Sugar: 1g

Stuffed Acorn Squash and Cranberries

Prep Time: 15 minutes
Cooking Time: 40-45 minutes
Serving Size: 4

Ingredients

2 acorn squash, halved and seeds removed

1 cup cooked quinoa

1/2 cup dried cranberries

1/4 cup chopped nuts (such as walnuts or pecans)

2 tablespoons chopped fresh herbs (such as parsley or thyme)

Salt to taste

Coconut oil for roasting

Cooking Instructions

Heat the oven to 400°F (200°C). Coat the insides of the acorn squash halves with coconut oil and season with salt. Lay the halves, cut side down, on a baking sheet covered with parchment paper. Roast in the oven for 25 to 30 minutes, or until they are soft. Transfer the cooked quinoa, chopped nuts, dried cranberries, and fresh herbs into a mixing bowl. Adjust the seasoning with salt. When the squash halves are soft, take them out of the oven and carefully turn them over. Spoon the quinoa mixture into each half, making sure to pack it in tightly.

Place the filled squash halves back into the oven and bake for a further ten to fifteen minutes, or until they are thoroughly heated and have a crunchy top.

Nutritional Values (per serving):
Calories: 250 kcal, Protein: 5g, Carbs: 45g, Fat: 7g, Fiber: 7g, Sugar: 10g

Chapter 4: Poultry, Meat and Potatoes AIP Recipes

Chicken Breast

Prep Time: 5 minutes
Cooking Time: 12-25 minutes
Serving Size: 4

Ingredients

4 boneless, skinless chicken breasts

2 tablespoons coconut oil or olive oil

Salt to taste

AIP-friendly herbs and spices (e.g., garlic powder, onion powder, dried thyme)

Cooking Instructions

To ensure that your chicken breasts don't stick, brush them with oil before grilling them for 6-7 minutes on each side, or until they reach an internal temperature of 165°F (75°C). If you're using an oven, skillet, or grill, preheat the heat to medium-high. Pat the chicken breasts dry with paper towels and season both sides with salt and AIP-friendly herbs and spices. To bake: Preheat your oven to 400°F (200°C). Arrange the seasoned chicken breasts on a baking sheet lined with parchment paper. Bake for 20 to 25 minutes, or until the chicken reaches an internal temperature of 165°F (75°C). Alternatively, you can sauté the chicken by heating coconut oil or olive oil in a skillet over medium-high heat.

After the chicken is cooked through and has a golden brown exterior, remove it from the heat source.

Nutritional Values (per serving 4 oz cooked chicken breast):
Calories: 150 kca, Protein: 30g, Fat: 3g, Sodium: 60mg

Turkey Thighs

Prep Time: 10 minutes
Cooking Time: 1½ to 2 hours
Serving Size: 4

Ingredients

4 turkey thighs, bone-in and skin removed

2 tablespoons coconut oil

2 teaspoons dried thyme

2 teaspoons dried oregano

2 teaspoons garlic powder

Salt to taste

1 cup chicken or turkey broth

Cooking Instructions

In a small bowl, combine the dried thyme, dried oregano, garlic powder, and salt. Rub the spice mixture evenly over the turkey thighs. Preheat your oven to 325°F (163°C). Warm up the coconut oil in a large skillet over medium-high heat. Add the turkey thighs to the skillet and brown on both sides, about 3–4 minutes per side. Transfer the browned turkey thighs to a baking dish. Fill the baking dish with chicken or turkey broth, cover with aluminum foil, and pop into the preheated oven. Bake the turkey thighs for one and a half to two hours, or until they are tender and cooked through.

Take the baking dish out of the oven and allow the turkey thighs to rest for a few minutes before serving.

Duck Breast

Prep Time: 5 minutes
Cooking Time: 10-12 minutes
Serving Size: 2

Ingredients

2 duck breasts

Salt to taste

AIP-friendly herbs and spices (such as thyme, rosemary, and garlic powder)

Cooking Instructions

Preheat a skillet over medium-high heat. Score the duck breasts' skin in a crisscross pattern, being careful not to cut into the meat. Season the duck breasts on both sides with salt and your preferred AIP-friendly herbs and spices. Place the duck breasts skin-side down in the skillet and cook for 5 to 7 minutes, until the skin is golden brown and crispy. After a few minutes, turn the duck breasts over and cook for a further three to five minutes, or until done to your liking. Take the duck breasts out of the skillet and allow them to cool before slicing.

Nutritional Values (per serving):
Calories: 250 kcal, Protein: 20g, Carbs: 0g, Fat: 18g, Fiber: 0g, Sugar: 0g

Cornish Hen

Prep Time: 10 minutes
Cooking Time: 60-75 minutes
Serving Size: 2 servings

Ingredients

2 Cornish hens

2 tablespoons coconut oil, melted

2 teaspoons dried thyme

2 teaspoons dried oregano

2 teaspoons garlic powder

Salt to taste

Cooking Instructions

Preheat the oven to 375°F (190°C). Rinse the hens under cold water and pat dry with paper towels. In a small bowl, combine the melted coconut oil, dried thyme, dried oregano, garlic powder, and salt. Rub the herb mixture all over the hens, making sure to coat them evenly. A roasting pan or baking dish should be used for the Cornish hens. Roast in the preheated oven for approximately 60–75 minutes, or until the internal temperature reaches 165°F (74°C) when measured with a meat thermometer inserted into the thickest part of the hen. Once cooked, remove the Cornish hens from the oven and allow them to rest for 5–10 minutes before serving.

Nutritional Values (per serving):
Calories: 400 kcal, Protein: 40g, Carbs: 0g, Fat: 26g, Fiber: 0g, Sugar: 0g

Quail

Prep Time: 10 minutes
Cooking Time: 25-30 minutes
Serving Size: 4

Ingredients

4 whole quails, cleaned

2 tablespoons coconut oil

2 cloves garlic, minced

1 teaspoon dried thyme

Salt to taste

Cooking Instructions

Set the oven to 375°F (190°C). Combine the minced garlic, dried thyme, and salt in a small bowl. Apply coconut oil to the quails, then evenly coat them with the herb mixture. Transfer the quails to an oven-safe skillet or roasting pan. Roast in the preheated oven for 25 to 30 minutes, or until the quails are cooked through and golden brown, basting them occasionally with the pan juices. Remove from the oven and let the quails rest for a few minutes before serving.

Nutritional Values (per serving):
Calories: 180 kcal, Protein: 25g, Carbs: 0g, Fat: 8g, Cholesterol: 95mg, Sodium: 65mg

Beef Chuck Roast

Prep Time: 15 minutes
Cooking Time: 2½ -3 hours
Serving Size: 4-6

Ingredients

2-3 lbs beef chuck roast

2 tablespoons coconut oil or olive oil

1 onion, sliced

3 cloves garlic, minced

2 carrots, chopped

2 celery stalks, chopped

1 cup bone broth or beef broth (check for AIP-compliant ingredients)

2 bay leaves

1 teaspoon dried thyme

Salt to taste

Cooking Instructions

Preheat your oven to 325°F (160°C). In a Dutch oven or oven-safe pot, heat up some coconut oil or olive oil over medium-high heat. Sear the beef chuck roast on all sides until browned, about 3-4 minutes per side. Remove the roast from the pot and set aside. Add the chopped onion, minced garlic, chopped carrots, and chopped celery, and cook for 5 to 7 minutes, or until the vegetables begin to soften.

Return the roast to the pot, add the bone broth or beef broth, bay leaves, dried thyme, and salt to taste. Cover the pot with a lid and place it in the preheated oven; cook for 2.5 to 3 hours, or until the beef is tender and easily pulls apart with a fork. Once cooked, remove the pot from the oven and let it rest for a few minutes before serving. Serve the beef chuck roast hot, sliced or shredded, with the vegetables and juices from the pot.

Nutritional Values (per serving):
Calories: 350 kcal, Protein: 30g, Carbs: 6g, Fat: 23g, Fiber: 1g, Sugar: 2g

Lamb Chops

Prep Time: 5 minutes
Cooking Time: 8-10 minutes
Serving Size: 2

Ingredients

4 lamb chops

2 tablespoons coconut oil

2 cloves garlic, minced (optional, omit if sensitive)

1 teaspoon dried rosemary

1 teaspoon dried thyme

Salt to taste

Cooking Instructions

Combine salt, dried thyme, and rosemary in a small bowl. Apply the herb mixture evenly to the lamb chops on both sides. Heat coconut oil in a skillet over medium-high heat. Add the lamb chops and sear for 3–4 minutes on each side, or until done to your liking. Remove the lamb chops from the skillet and let rest for a few minutes before serving; if using minced garlic, add it to the skillet during the last minute of cooking, stirring constantly to avoid burning.

Nutritional Values (per serving):
Calories: 300 kcal, Protein: 22g, Carbs: 0g, Fat: 23g, Fiber: 0g, Sugar: 0g

Pork Tenderloin

Prep Time: 10 minutes (plus marinating time)
Cooking Time: 25-30 minutes
Serving Size: 4

Ingredients

1 lb pork tenderloin

2 tablespoons apple cider vinegar

2 tablespoons coconut aminos

2 cloves garlic, minced

1 teaspoon dried thyme

1 teaspoon dried rosemary

1/2 teaspoon sea salt

1/4 teaspoon black pepper (optional, omit for strict AIP)

Cooking Instructions

Whisk together the coconut aminos, minced garlic, dried thyme, dried rosemary, sea salt, and black pepper in a small bowl. Transfer the pork tenderloin to a shallow dish or resealable plastic bag, making sure the tenderloin is well coated with the marinade. Marinate for a minimum of 30 minutes, or up to 4 hours, for the most flavor. Set your oven to 400°F (200°C).

Take the pork tenderloin out of the marinade and throw away any extra marinade. Transfer the pork tenderloin to a baking dish or a parchment paper-lined baking sheet. Roast the pork tenderloin for 25 to 30 minutes, rotating it halfway through, or until the internal temperature reaches 145°F (63°C). After cooking, take the pork tenderloin out of the oven and allow it to rest for 5 minutes before slicing.

Nutritional Values (per serving):
Calories: 180 kcal, Protein: 25g, Carbs: 2g, Fat: 7g, Fiber: 0g, Sugar: 0g

Venison

Prep Time: 10 minutes
Cooking Time: 20-25 minutes
Serving Size: 4

Ingredients

1 lb venison, preferably a tender cut like loin or tenderloin

2 tablespoons coconut oil or avocado oil

2 cloves garlic, minced (optional, omit if sensitive)

1 teaspoon dried thyme

1 teaspoon dried rosemary

Salt to taste

Cooking Instructions

Pat the venison dry with paper towels and season generously with salt. In a small bowl, combine the coconut oil or avocado oil, minced garlic, dried thyme, and dried rosemary to make a seasoning mixture. Rub the seasoning mixture all over the venison, making sure it's evenly coated. Preheat your oven to 375°F (190°C). In a roasting pan or oven-safe skillet, place the seasoned venison. Roast in the preheated oven for about 20 to 25 minutes for medium-rare, or until an internal meat thermometer reads 135°F (57°C). After taking the venison out of the oven, let it rest for 5 to 10 minutes before slicing. Serve the venison hot, thinly sliced against the grain.

Nutritional Values (per serving):
Calories: 180 kcal, Protein: 25g, Carbs: 0g, Fat: 9g, Fiber: 0g, Sugar: 0g

Buffalo/Bison

Prep Time: 10 minutes
Cooking Time: 15 minutes
Serving Size: 4

Ingredients

1 lb bison meat, thinly sliced

2 tablespoons coconut oil

3 cloves garlic, minced

1 tablespoon grated ginger

2 cups sliced vegetables (such as bell peppers, carrots, and broccoli)

2 tablespoons coconut aminos

Salt to taste

Optional: chopped green onions for garnish

Cooking Instructions

Heat the coconut oil in a large skillet or wok over medium-high heat. Add the grated ginger and minced garlic and cook for 1 to 2 minutes until fragrant. Cook the bison meat thinly sliced for 2 to 3 minutes until browned. Add the sliced vegetables and stir-fry for 5 to 7 minutes, or until they begin to soften. Add the coconut aminos to the stir-fry and cook for an additional two to three minutes, or until everything is well combined and heated through.

Taste and add salt as needed. You can also garnish with chopped green onions if you like.

Nutritional Values (per serving):
Calories: 250 kcal, Protein: 25g, Carbs: 8g, Fat: 13g, Fiber: 2g, Sugar: 3g

Sweet Potatoes

Prep Time: 10 minutes
Cooking Time: 25-30 minutes
Serving Size: 4

Ingredients

4 medium sweet potatoes

2 tablespoons coconut oil, melted

Salt to taste

Optional: AIP-friendly herbs or spices like garlic powder, onion powder, or thyme

Cooking Instructions

Set the oven to 400°F (200°C). Scrub and wash the sweet potatoes under running water to get rid of any dirt. Peel and cut the sweet potatoes into cubes or wedges, depending on your choice. Transfer the sweet potatoes to a big mixing bowl and coat them evenly with melted coconut oil. Season with salt and any optional AIP-friendly herbs or spices. Spread the sweet potatoes in a single layer on a baking sheet lined with parchment paper or aluminum foil. Roast in the preheated oven for 25 to 30 minutes, or until the sweet potatoes are tender and lightly browned, flipping halfway through cooking. Once cooked, remove from the oven and let cool slightly before serving.

Nutritional Values (per serving):
Calories: 150 kcal, Protein: 2g, Carbs: 26g, Fat: 5g, Fiber: 4g, Sugar: 6g

Japanese Sweet Potatoes

Prep Time: 5 minutes
Cooking Time: 45-60 minutes
Serving Size: 4

Ingredients

4 Japanese sweet potatoes

Cooking Instructions

Set the oven to 400°F (200°C). Rinse and pat dry the Japanese sweet potatoes. Prick each one several times with a fork to release steam while cooking. Transfer the potatoes to a baking sheet covered with aluminum foil or parchment paper. Bake the sweet potatoes in the preheated oven for 45 to 60 minutes, or until a fork inserted into them pierces them easily.

Nutritional Values (per serving):
Calories: 130 kcal, Protein: 2g, Carbs: 30g, Fat: 0g, Fiber: 4g, Sugar: 6g

White Potatoes

Prep Time: 10 minutes
Cooking Time: 15-20 minutes
Serving Size: 4

Ingredients

4 medium-sized white potatoes, peeled and cubed

Water for boiling

Salt (optional)

Cooking Instructions

After peeling and chopping the white potatoes into uniform-sized cubes, put the cubed potatoes in a big pot with water, and if you want, add a pinch of salt. Bring the water to a boil over high heat, then lower the heat to medium-low and simmer the potatoes until they are tender, about 15 to 20 minutes. After that time, drain the potatoes in a colander. When it comes to potatoes, they can be served hot as a side dish or used as a foundation for other AIP-friendly toppings or sauces. For mashed potatoes, drain the potatoes and place them in a mixing bowl. Use a fork or potato masher to mash the potatoes until they're smooth. If you want to make them extra creamy, you can add a little bit of coconut milk or olive oil.

Nutritional Values (per serving, boiled potatoes):
Calories: 100 kcal, Protein: 2g, Carbs: 23g, Fat: 0g, Fiber: 2g, Sugar: 1g

Nutritional Values (per serving, mashed potatoes):
Calories: 120 kcal, Protein: 2g, Carbs: 26g, Fat: 1g, Fiber: 3g, Sugar: 1g

Yuca

Prep Time: 10 minutes
Cooking Time: 20-30 minutes
Serving Size: 4

Ingredients

1 large yuca root (cassava)

Water for boiling

Salt to taste

Cooking Instructions

After removing any tough or woody parts from the yuca root, peel it and cut it into chunks or slices. Rinse the yuca pieces under cold water to get rid of any dirt or debris. Bring a pot of salted water to a boil over high heat, add the yuca pieces, and cook for 20 to 30 minutes, or until the yuca is fork-tender. Once cooked, drain and transfer to a serving dish. You can mash or fry the yuca for a creamy or crispy texture, or serve hot as a side dish.

Nutritional Values (per serving, boiled yuca):
Calories: 220 kcal, Carbs: 55g, Fiber: 3g, Protein: 2g, Fat: 0g, Vitamin C: 42mg, Potassium: 558mg

Boiled Taro Root

Prep Time: 10 minutes
Cooking Time: 20-25 minutes
Serving Size: 4

Ingredients

2 medium taro roots

Water

Salt (optional)

Cooking Instructions

After peeling and cutting the taro roots into chunks or cubes, put the pieces in a pot with water, and optionally add a pinch of salt. Bring the water to a boil, then lower the heat and simmer the taro roots until they are soft to the touch when pierced with a fork. Once the taro roots are cooked, drain them and serve hot as a side dish or use them in other AIP recipes.

Nutritional Values (per serving):
Calories: 160 kcal, Protein: 2g, Carbs: 36g, Fat: 0g, Fiber: 4g, Sugar: 2g

Chapter 5: Sauces, Condiments and Dressings

Homemade Basil Pesto

Prep Time: 10 minutes
Cooking Time: 0 minutes
Serving Size: 1 cup of pesto

Ingredients

2 cups fresh basil leaves, packed

1/2 cup extra virgin olive oil

1/4 cup coconut cream

2 cloves garlic, minced (optional, omit if sensitive)

1 tablespoon lemon juice

Salt to taste

Cooking Instructions

Clean the basil leaves well and pat dry with paper towels. Put the basil leaves, extra virgin olive oil, coconut cream, minced garlic (if using), and lemon juice in a food processor or blender. Blend until smooth and well combined, scraping down the sides of the bowl as needed. Taste and add salt to taste, blending again to incorporate. Transfer the pesto to a jar or container that fits tightly and refrigerate until needed.

Nutritional Values (per serving - 1 tablespoon):
Calories: 70 kcal, Protein: 1g, Carbs: 1g, Fat: 7g, Fiber: 0g, Sugar: 0g

Coconut Aminos

Prep Time: 5 minutes
Cooking Time: 30-40 minutes
Serving Size: 1 cup

Ingredients

2 cups coconut water

2 tablespoons coconut sugar

1/2 teaspoon sea salt

Cooking Instructions

Coconut water, coconut sugar, and sea salt should all be combined in a small saucepan. The mixture should be brought to a simmer over medium heat, with occasional stirring to dissolve the coconut sugar. After the sugar is dissolved, the heat should be turned down to a low simmer for 30 to 40 minutes, or until the mixture has reduced by half and is syrupy. After turning off the heat and allowing the coconut aminos to cool completely, transfer them to a glass bottle or jar with a tight-fitting lid and keep them in the fridge for up to two weeks.

Nutritional Values (per tablespoon serving):
Calories: 20 kcal, Carbs: 5g, Sugars: 4g

Tahini Dressing

Prep Time: 5 minutes
Serving Size: 4 servings

Ingredients

1/4 cup tahini

2 tablespoons lemon juice

2 tablespoons apple cider vinegar

2 tablespoons extra virgin olive oil

1 clove garlic, minced (optional, omit if sensitive)

2-4 tablespoons water, to thin

Salt to taste

Cooking Instructions

In a small mixing bowl, whisk together tahini, lemon juice, apple cider vinegar, olive oil, and minced garlic (if using). Gradually add water, 1 tablespoon at a time, until the dressing reaches your desired consistency; the amount of water may need to be adjusted depending on how thick your tahini is. Season with salt to taste. Whisk until smooth. Serve over salads, roasted vegetables, or grilled meats.

Nutritional Values (per serving):
Calories: 120 kcal, Protein: 2g, Carbs: 4g, Fat: 11g, Fiber: 1g, Sugar: 0g

Garlic-Herb Aioli

Prep Time: 5 minutes
Serving Size: 1/2 cup of aioli

Ingredients

1/2 cup coconut cream (chilled)

2 tablespoons extra virgin olive oil

1 tablespoon apple cider vinegar

2 cloves garlic, minced (omit if sensitive to garlic)

1 tablespoon chopped fresh herbs (such as parsley, basil, or cilantro)

Salt to taste

Cooking Instructions

In a small mixing bowl, combine the chilled coconut cream, extra virgin olive oil, and apple cider vinegar. Whisk until smooth and well combined. Stir in the minced garlic (if using) and chopped fresh herbs. Season with salt to taste and mix until well combined. Cover and refrigerate the aioli for at least 30 minutes to allow the flavors to meld together. Serve chilled as a dip or spread for meats, veggies, or seafood.

Nutritional Values (per serving 2 tablespoons):
Calories: 120 kcal, Protein: 1g, Carbs: 3g, Fat: 12g, Fiber: 0g, Sugar: 1g

Avocado Lime Dressing

Prep Time: 5 minutes
Serving Size: 6 servings

Ingredients

1 ripe avocado, peeled and pitted

1/4 cup fresh lime juice

2 tablespoons extra virgin olive oil

2 tablespoons chopped fresh cilantro

1 clove garlic, minced (optional, omit if sensitive)

Salt to taste

Water (as needed to adjust consistency)

Cooking Instructions

Combine the avocado, lime juice, olive oil, cilantro, and minced garlic in a blender or food processor. Blend until smooth and creamy. If the dressing is too thick, you can add a little water, one tablespoon at a time, until you reach your desired consistency. Taste and adjust the seasoning with salt as needed. Transfer the dressing to a jar or container with a tight-fitting lid. Store in the refrigerator for up to three to four days.

Nutritional Values (per serving):
Calories: 80 kcal, Protein: 1g, Carbs: 4g, Fat: 7g, Fiber: 3g, Sugar: 0g

Cilantro Lime Chimichurri

Prep Time: 5 minutes
Serving Size: 1 cup

Ingredients

1 cup fresh cilantro, chopped

2 cloves garlic, minced (omit if following strict AIP)

1/4 cup extra virgin olive oil

2 tablespoons lime juice

1/2 teaspoon apple cider vinegar

Salt to taste

Cooking Instructions

Chopped cilantro, minced garlic, extra virgin olive oil, lime juice, and apple cider vinegar should all be combined in a food processor or blender. Pulse until the mixture reaches your desired consistency; it can be blended until smooth or left slightly chunky. Season with salt to taste, adjusting the acidity of the lime juice or vinegar if needed. Transfer the chimichurri to a serving bowl or jar.

Nutritional Values (per serving, based on 2 tablespoons):
Calories: 120 kcal, Protein: 0g, Carbs: 1g, Fat: 14g, Fiber: 0g, Sugar: 0g

Apple Cider Vinaigrette

Prep Time: 5 minutes
Serving Size: 8 servings

Ingredients

1/2 cup apple cider vinegar

1/4 cup extra virgin olive oil

1 tablespoon raw honey (optional, omit if avoiding sweeteners)

1 teaspoon minced garlic

1 teaspoon grated fresh ginger

1/2 teaspoon sea salt

1/4 teaspoon ground black pepper (optional, omit for AIP compliance)

Cooking Instructions

In a small bowl or glass jar, whisk together apple cider vinegar, extra virgin olive oil, raw honey (if using), minced garlic, grated fresh ginger, sea salt, and ground black pepper (if using). Continue whisking until the ingredients are well combined and the vinaigrette is smooth. Taste and adjust seasoning, adding more salt or honey. Serve immediately or store in an airtight container in the refrigerator for up to 1 week. Shake well before serving.

Nutritional Values (per serving):
Calories: 80 kcal, Protein: 0g, Carbs: 2g, Fat: 9g, Fiber: 0g, Sugar: 2g

Carrot Ginger Dressing

Prep Time: 10 minutes
Serving Size: 8 servings

Ingredients

2 medium carrots, peeled and roughly chopped

1-inch piece of fresh ginger, peeled and grated

2 tablespoons apple cider vinegar

2 tablespoons extra virgin olive oil

2 tablespoons water

1 tablespoon coconut aminos

1 tablespoon honey (optional, omit for strict AIP)

Salt to taste

Cooking Instructions

Grated ginger, chopped carrots, apple cider vinegar, olive oil, water, coconut aminos, and honey (if using) should all be combined in a blender or food processor and blended until smooth and well combined. You can adjust the dressing's consistency by adding a little more water if necessary. Taste and adjust the seasoning with salt if necessary. Transfer the dressing to a sealed container and refrigerate for at least 30 minutes to allow the flavors to meld together. Shake well before serving.

Nutritional Values (per serving):
Calories: 35 kcal, Protein: 0.3g, Carbs: 3g, Fat: 2.5g,Fiber: 0.6g, Sugar: 1.6g

Lemon Herb Marinade

Prep Time: 10 minutes
Serving Size: 4

Ingredients

1/4 cup fresh lemon juice

2 tablespoons extra virgin olive oil

2 cloves garlic, minced

1 tablespoon fresh parsley, finely chopped

1 tablespoon fresh thyme leaves, finely chopped

1 tablespoon fresh rosemary, finely chopped

Salt to taste

Cooking Instructions

 In a small bowl, whisk together the lemon juice, olive oil, minced garlic, chopped parsley, chopped thyme, and chopped rosemary. Season with salt to taste and mix well to combine.
Use the marinade right away or store it in the refrigerator for up to three days in an airtight container.

Nutritional Values (per serving, marinade only):
Calories: 50 kcal, Protein: 0g, Carbs: 2g, Fat: 5g, Fiber: 0g, Sugar: 0g

Onion Ginger Sauce

Prep Time: 5 minutes
Serving Size: 4 servings

Ingredients

4 green onions, finely chopped

1 tablespoon fresh ginger, grated

2 tablespoons coconut aminos

1 tablespoon apple cider vinegar

1 tablespoon olive oil

1 tablespoon water

Salt to taste

Cooking Instructions

In a small bowl, combine chopped green onions, grated ginger, coconut aminos, apple cider vinegar, olive oil, and water. Stir until well combined. Taste and adjust seasoning with salt if necessary. Let the sauce sit for 10 to 15 minutes to allow the flavors to meld. Serve as a dipping sauce or drizzle over cooked meats, seafood, or vegetables.

Nutritional Values (per serving):
Calories: 35 kcal, Protein: 1g, Carbs: 3g, Fat: 2g, Fiber: 1g, Sugar: 1g

Chapter 6: Drinks and Teas AIP Recipes

Bone Broth

Prep Time: 15 minutes
Cooking Time: 12-24 hours
Serving Size: 8-10 cups

Ingredients

2-3 lbs of grass-fed beef bones or pasture-raised chicken bones

2 carrots, chopped

2 celery stalks, chopped

1 onion, chopped

4 cloves garlic, smashed

2 tablespoons apple cider vinegar

Water, enough to cover the bones

Salt to taste

Cooking Instructions

After preheating the oven to 400°F (200°C), put the bones on a baking sheet and roast them for about 30 minutes, or until they are nicely browned. Then, transfer the roasted bones to a large stockpot or slow cooker, cover the bones completely with water, and add chopped carrots, celery, onion, garlic, and apple cider vinegar. Bring the mixture to a boil over high heat, then reduce the heat to low and let it simmer gently for 12 to 24 hours.

The longer you simmer the mixture, the richer and more flavorful the broth will be. Skim off any foam or impurities that rise to the surface during cooking. After the broth has finished simmering, strain it through a fine mesh sieve or cheesecloth to remove the bones and vegetables, then discard the solids. After allowing the broth to cool, pour it into jars or other storage containers and refrigerate for up to five days. Alternatively, freeze the broth for extended storage.

Nutritional Values (per serving,1 cup):
Calories: 45 kcal, Protein: 5g, Carbs: 2g, Fat: 2g, Fiber: 0g, Sugar: 1g

Peppermint Tea

Prep Time: 1 minute
Cooking Time: 5-7 minutes
Serving Size: 2

Ingredients

1 tablespoon dried peppermint leaves

2 cups water

Cooking Instructions

After bringing two cups of water to a boil in a kettle or saucepan, add the dried peppermint leaves to a teapot or other heat-resistant container, cover the peppermint leaves with boiling water, and let steep for five to seven minutes, allowing the flavor of the peppermint to seep into the water. Finally, strain the tea into cups or mugs.

Ginger Tea

Prep Time: 5 minutes
Cooking Time: 10-15 minutes
Serving Size: 2-4

Ingredients

1-2 inches fresh ginger root, thinly sliced or grated

4 cups filtered water

Optional: Honey (in moderation, if tolerated) or lemon juice for flavor

Cooking Instructions

In a small saucepan, bring the filtered water to a boil. Add the thinly sliced or grated ginger root to the boiling water. Reduce the heat to low and let the ginger simmer in the water for about 10-15 minutes, depending on how strong the flavor you want. Assemble the ginger pieces and strain the tea; pour the ginger tea into mugs and serve hot. You can optionally add a drizzle of honey or a squeeze of lemon juice for extra flavor.

Chamomile Tea

Prep Time: 1 minute
Cooking Time: 5-10 minutes
Serving Size: 1 cup

Ingredients

2 teaspoons dried chamomile flowers

1 cup boiling water

Cooking Instructions

After adding the boiling water to the dried chamomile flowers in a heatproof mug or teapot, cover and steep for five to ten minutes to allow the flavors to infuse. Strain the tea to remove the chamomile flowers.

Dandelion Root Tea

Prep Time: 5 minutes
Cooking Time: 15-20 minutes
Serving Size: 4 cups

Ingredients

2 tablespoons dried dandelion roots (make sure they are harvested from a pesticide-free area)

4 cups water

Cooking Instructions

After washing the dried dandelion roots in cold water to get rid of any dirt or debris, put 4 cups of water in a medium saucepan, add the dried dandelion roots, and boil the water for 10 to 15 minutes. Then, take the saucepan off the heat and let the tea steep for an additional 5 to 10 minutes. Strain the tea to get rid of the dandelion roots, then pour the hot tea into cups

Rooibos Tea

Prep Time: (while water is boiling)
Cooking Time: 5-7 minutes
Serving Size: 2

Ingredients

2 cups water

2-3 rooibos tea bags

Cooking Instructions

In a saucepan, bring two cups of water to a boil. Once boiling, remove from the heat and add the rooibos tea bags. Steep the tea bags in the hot water for five to seven minutes, depending on the strength you want. Then, remove and discard the tea bags and pour the brewed rooibos tea into serving cups.

Coconut Water

Prep Time: 5 minutes
Serving Size: 2 cups of coconut water

Ingredients

1 fresh coconut (green, not mature)

Filtered water

Cooking Instructions

Start by choosing a fresh green coconut, being careful not to choose one that is mature, as mature coconuts have thicker flesh and less water. Use a sturdy knife to carefully chop off the top of the coconut, creating a small opening to access the water inside. Pour the coconut water into a clean glass or container, straining it through a fine mesh sieve if necessary.

Nutritional Values (per serving - 1 cup):
Calories: 45 kcal, Carbs: 9g, Protein: 2g, Fat: 0g, Fiber: 3g Sugar: 6g

Turmeric Latte

Prep Time: 5 minutes
Cooking Time: 5 minutes
Serving Size: 2

Ingredients

2 cups coconut milk (or any other AIP-friendly milk alternative)

1 teaspoon ground turmeric

1/2 teaspoon ground cinnamon

1/4 teaspoon ground ginger

Pinch of ground black pepper (optional, omit if sensitive)

1 tablespoon honey or maple syrup (optional, for sweetness)

Cooking Instructions

Heat the coconut milk in a small saucepan over medium heat, without bringing it to a boil. Whisk in the ground turmeric, ginger, cinnamon, and black pepper. Allow the flavors to mingle for two to three minutes, stirring occasionally. Taste and adjust the sweetness by adding honey or maple syrup, if desired, and stirring until dissolved. Take the mixture off the heat and pour the turmeric latte into mugs.

Nutritional Values (per serving):
Calories: 150 kcal, Protein: 1g, Carbs: 4g, Fat: 14g, Fiber: 1g, Sugar: 3g

Fruit Infused Water

Prep Time: 5 minutes
Infusing Time: 2 hours or overnight
Serving Size: 4

Ingredients

1 liter of filtered water

1 cup of mixed fruits (such as sliced strawberries, sliced oranges, and sliced cucumber)

Cooking Instructions

The mixed fruits should be combined in a large pitcher, then covered and chilled for at least two hours or overnight to allow the flavors to infuse. Serve chilled over ice. Pour filtered water over the fruits and gently stir to combine.

28 DAYS MEAL PLAN

Week 1

- Day 1: AIP Breakfast Skillet

- Day 2: Chicken and Vegetable Stir-Fry

- Day 3: Turmeric Scrambled Eggs

- Day 4: Coconut Berry Bliss Balls

- Day 5: Roasted Sweet Potato and Kale Salad

- Day 6: Stuffed Bell Peppers

- Day 7: Sweet Potato Hash

Week 2

- Day 8: AIP Trail Mix

- Day 9: Cauliflower Rice Stir-Fry

- Day 10: Baked Apples with Cinnamon

- Day 11: Buffalo/Bison

- Day 12: Coconut Flour Pancakes

- Day 13: Portobello Mushroom Burgers

- Day 14: Turmeric Latte

Week 3

- Day 15: AIP Breakfast Burrito Bowl

- Day 16: Grilled Eggplant with Balsamic Glaze

- Day 17: Baked Acorn Squash with Cinnamon

- Day 18: Duck Breast

- Day 19: Coconut Water

- Day 20: Butternut Squash Soup

- Day 21: Lemon Herb Marinade

Week 4

- Day 22: AIP Breakfast Casserole

- Day 23: Cabbage Rolls with Cauliflower Rice

- Day 24: Baked Sweet Potato Chips

- Day 25: Pork Tenderloin

- Day 26: Coconut Aminos

- Day 27: Sweet Potatoes

- Day 28: Apple Cider Vinaigrette

Feel free to shuffle the days or repeat any recipes based on your preferences and nutritional needs.

Recommended Supplements to Support Healing

Although the Autoimmune Protocol (AIP) diet emphasizes whole foods high in nutrients to promote healing and lower inflammation, adding specific supplements can help those who suffer from autoimmune diseases. These supplements can support immune function and improve gut health, among other things.

1 Probiotics

- Role: Probiotics are good bacteria that boost immunity and maintain a balanced microbiome to support gut health.

- Benefits: Supplementing with probiotics has been linked to better digestion, lowered inflammatory levels, and strengthened immune function.

- Recommended Form: Seek out premium probiotic supplements with a range of strains, such as Bifidobacterium and Lactobacillus species.

2. Digestive Enzymes

- Role: In order to promote optimal digestion and nutrient assimilation, digestive enzymes help break down and absorb nutrients from foods.

- Benefits: Digestive enzyme supplements can improve nutrient absorption and reduce digestive discomfort, including gas and bloating, especially in people with impaired gut health.

- Recommended Form: Select a broad-spectrum digestive enzyme supplement that aids in the breakdown of proteins, fats, and carbohydrates by including lipases, amylases, and proteases.

3 Omega-3 Fatty Acids

- Role: The anti-inflammatory qualities of omega-3 fatty acids, especially those of eicosapentaenoic acid (EPA) and docosahexaenoic acid (DHA), promote cardiovascular and mental health.

- Benefits: Omega-3 fatty acid supplements can help lower inflammation, maintain joint health, and enhance mood stability and brain function.

- Recommended Form: To get the bioactive forms of omega-3 fatty acids, EPA and DHA, think about taking supplements made of algae or fish oil.

4 Collagen

- Role: The primary structural protein in the body, collagen is necessary to keep the skin, bones, and connective tissues intact.

- Benefits: Collagen supplements can improve joint function and mobility, support gut health, and encourage skin elasticity and hydration

- Recommended Form: Select hydrolyzed collagen supplements for supporting gut health and tissue repair, as they are highly bioavailable and easily digestible.

5 Vitamin D

- Role: An essential vitamin for immune system function, healthy bones, and general wellbeing is vitamin D

- Benefits: Vitamin D supplements can help the body's defenses against disease, lessen inflammation, and increase the body's ability to absorb calcium and form bones.

- Recommended Form: Rather than taking vitamin D2 supplements, choose vitamin D3 supplements since they are more bioactive and efficient at increasing the body's vitamin D levels.

6 Magnesium

- Role: The body uses magnesium as a necessary mineral for hundreds of enzymatic processes, including the synthesis of energy, the contraction of muscles, and the transmission of nerve signals.

- Benefits: Magnesium supplements can improve sleep quality and relaxation, reduce cramping in the muscles, and control blood pressure and sugar levels

- Recommended Form: Select magnesium malate, glycinate, or citrate for maximum bioavailability and absorption.

7 L-Glutamine

- Role: One amino acid that is essential for preserving the integrity of the intestinal lining and promoting the function of the gut barrier is glutamine.

- Benefits: By reducing intestinal permeability (leaky gut), repairing and healing the gut lining, and easing the symptoms of digestive disorders, L-glutamine supplements can help.

- Recommended Form: To support gut health, look for L-glutamine powder or capsules that are easy to take as a supplement and think about including it in your daily routine.

8 Turmeric/Curcumin

- Role: Curcumin, a strong anti-inflammatory substance with antioxidant qualities that boost immune system performance and lessen inflammation, is found in turmeric

- Benefits: Taking supplements containing turmeric or curcumin can support joint health, ease pain and inflammation brought on by autoimmune diseases, and enhance general wellbeing

- Recommended Form: To improve absorption and bioavailability, choose standardized curcumin supplements that also contain piperine, or black pepper extract.

9 Zinc

- Role: Zinc is a necessary mineral for DNA synthesis, wound healing, and immune system function

- Benefits: Zinc supplements can improve wound healing, lower inflammation, strengthen the immune system, and improve skin health

- Recommended Form: Instead of taking zinc oxide supplements, choose zinc picolinate or zinc citrate, as they are more readily absorbed and have fewer adverse effects on the gastrointestinal tract.

10 Vitamin C

- Role: Strong antioxidant vitamin C promotes tissue repair, collagen synthesis, and immunological function

- Benefits: Taking vitamin C supplements can improve wound healing, lower oxidative stress, strengthen the immune system, and support healthy skin

- Recommended Form: For the best absorption and bioavailability, select vitamin C supplements that contain ascorbic acid, calcium ascorbate, or magnesium ascorbate.

N.B *Choose high-quality supplements from reliable brands to ensure purity, potency, and safety. Keep in mind that supplements are meant to supplement, not replace, a nutrient-rich diet and lifestyle. Think about introducing supplements gradually and monitoring your body's response to ensure tolerability and efficacy.*

Transitioning Off AIP: Reintroduction Phase

You may eventually reach a point where you're ready to reintroduce certain foods back into your diet as you make progress on your AIP journey and notice improvements in your overall health and symptoms. The reintroduction phase gives you the opportunity to determine your specific dietary sensitivity and create a personalized, sustainable eating plan.

1. Reintroduce one food at a time in small amounts, starting with less likely to cause reactions. Observe how your body reacts to the food, both right away and in the hours and days that follow

2. After reintroducing a particular food, note any symptoms or mood swings you experience. Common reactions include headaches, fatigue, joint pain, rashes, and stomach problems.

3. Observe whether a food that has been reintroduced causes symptoms or reactions, record the intensity and duration of any reactions, and decide if it is worth reintroducing the food in the future based on your findings.

4. Focus on developing a customized approach to eating that supports your health and well-being while allowing for flexibility and enjoyment. Based on your findings during the reintroduction phase, modify your diet to exclude or limit foods that cause adverse reactions.

INDEX

Coconut Flour Pancakes 14

Coconut Water 107
Cornish Hen 71
Crispy Baked Plantain Chips 52
Cucumber Avocado Boats 37
Dandelion Root Tea 105
Duck Breast 70
Fruit Infused Water 109
Garlic-Herb Aioli 91
Ginger Tea 103
Grilled Eggplant with Balsamic Glaze 59
Homemade Basil Pesto 88
Japanese Sweet Potatoes 82
Lamb Chops 75
Lemon Herb Marinade 96
Mashed Turnips with Herbs 58
Noodles with Pesto 46
Onion Ginger Sauce 97
Peppermint Tea 102
Plantain Waffles 26
Pork Tenderloin 76
Portobello Mushroom Burgers 48
Quail 72
Roasted Sweet Potato and Kale Salad 42
Rooibos Tea 106
Smoked Salmon and Avocado Wrap 24
Spinach and Mushroom Avocado Dressing 61
Stuffed Acorn Squash and Cranberries 63
Stuffed Bell Peppers 49
Sweet Potatoes 81
Sweet Potato Hash 12
Tahini Dressing 90
Turmeric Coconut Porridge 29
Turmeric Scrambled Eggs 20
Turmeric Latte 108
Turkey Thighs 68
Venison 78

REFERENCES

About the Office of Autoimmune Disease Research (OADR-ORWH) | Office of Research on Women's Health. (n.d.). https://orwh.od.nih.gov/OADR-ORWH

Autoimmune Association. (2023, December 16). *Disease Information - Autoimmune Association.* https://autoimmune.org/disease-information/

Christovich, A., & Luo, X. (2022). Gut microbiota, leaky gut, and autoimmune diseases. *Frontiers in Immunology, 13.* https://doi.org/10.3389/.2022.946248

Clinic, C. (2024, March 29). *A little of this and that: Your guide to the AIP diet.* Cleveland Clinic. https://health.clevelandclinic.org/aip-diet-autoimmune-protocol-diet

Konijeti, G. G., Kim, N., Lewis, J. D., Groven, S., Chandrasekaran, A., Grandhe, S., Caroline, D., Singh, E., Oliveira, G., Wang, X., Molparia, B., & Torkamani, A. (2017). Efficacy of the autoimmune protocol diet for inflammatory bowel Disease. *Inflammatory Bowel Diseases*, *23*(11), 2054–2060. https://doi.org/10.1097/mib.0000000000001221

Mailing, L., PhD. (2020, July 5). *The evidence behind the autoimmune protocol diet (and how to try AIP)*. Lucy Mailing, PhD. https://www.lucymailing.com/ the evidence-behind the autoimmune protocol diet and how to try aip

Research Breakdown on Autoimmune Protocol (AIP) diet - examine. (n.d.). https://examine.com/diets/aip-diet/research/

Shaheen, W., Quraishi, M. N., & Iqbal, T. (2022). Gut microbiome and autoimmune disorders. *Clinical and Experimental Immunology (Print)*, *209*(2), 161–174. https://doi.org/10.1093/cei/uxac057

Wu, H., & Wu, E. (2012). The role of gut microbiota in immune homeostasis and autoimmunity. *Gut Microbes*, *3*(1), 4–14. https://doi.org/10.4161/gmic.19320

Printed in Great Britain
by Amazon

42140992R00076